Colour **Aids**

D0510069

Hand Conditions

Douglas W. Lamb MB ChB FRCSE

Consultant Orthopaedic Surgeon and
Surgeon in Charge of Hand Clinics at the
Royal Infirmary, Western General Hospital
and the Princess Margaret Rose Orthopaedic
Hospital, Edinburgh, UK

Geoffrey Hooper MMSc FRCS FRCSE

Senior Lecturer in Orthopaedic Surgery,
University of Edinburgh; Honorary
Consultant Orthopaedic Surgeon, Royal
Infirmary and Princess Margaret Rose
Orthopaedic Hospital, Edinburgh and
Bangour General Hospital, West Lothian, UK

Churchill Livingstone

EDINBURGH LONDON MELBOURNE AND NEW YORK 1984

Acknowledgements

We wish to thank: Professor S. P. F. Hughes who has allowed us to use material from the teaching slide collection in the Department of Orthopaedic Surgery, University of Edinburgh (Figs 3, 41, 67, 72, 75, 76, 87, 90, 95, 102, 129) and Professor J. A. A. Hunter who has provided us with slides from the collection in the Department of Dermatology, University of Edinburgh (Figs 88, 89, 122, 123, 135); Mr R. Bryson for Figs 50, 101; Mr C. Court-Brown for Fig. 132; Dr E. Housley for Figs 51, 125, 126, 127; Dr K. Little for Figs 79, 80; Mr M. Macnicol for Figs 58, 59; Mr Michael Devlin and Mr Graeme Ainslie of the Princess Margaret Rose Orthopaedic Hospital for their expert photography; Mrs Alison McGowan who has typed the manuscript.

Contents

Estelle M Holligan

1. **Complications of injury** 1
2. **Elevation and splintage** 3
3. **Fractures of the phalanges** 5
4. **Fractures of the metacarpal bones** 9
5. **Carpal injuries** 11
6. **Joint injuries** 13
7. **Tendon injuries** 17
8. **Nerve injuries** 23
9. **Finger tip injuries** 27
10. **Special types of injury** 31
11. **Self inflicted injuries** 35
12. **Finger amputations** 37
13. **Congenital anomalies** 41
    Failure of formation 41
    Failure of separation 43
    Duplication 43
    Overgrowth 45
    Constriction bands 45
    Miscellaneous 47
    Generalised skeletal abnormalities 49
14. **Hand infections** 53
    Pulp space 53
    Paronychia 53
    Web space 55
    Tendon sheath 55
    Septic arthritis 57
    Pyogenic granuloma 57
    Warts 59
    Orf 59
    Herpetic whitlow 59
    Erysipeloid 61
    Scabies 61
    Anthrax 63
    Leprosy 63

15. **Benign tumours** 65
    Ganglion 65
    Inclusion dermoid 65
    Lipoma 67
    Pigmented nodular synovitis 67
    Glomus tumour 69
    Aneurysm 69
    Enchondroma 71
    Exostosis 71
16. **Malignant tumours** 73
    Squamous carcinoma 73
    Malignant melanoma 73
    Chondrosarcoma 73
17. **Dupuytren's disease** 75
18. **Rheumatoid arthritis** 79
19. **Osteoarthritis** 87
    Heberden's nodes 87
    Mucous cyst 87
    Carpometacarpal joint of thumb 89
20. **Gout** 89
21. **Skin diseases** 91
    Psoriasis 91
    Eczema 93
    Vitiligo 93
22. **Circulatory disorders** 95
    Scleroderma 95
    Acrocyanosis 95
23. **Carpal tunnel syndrome** 97
24. **Stenosing tenosynovitis** 99
    De Quervain's tenosynovitis 99
    Trigger finger 99
25. **Volkmann's contracture** 101
26. **Cerebral palsy** 101
27. **Nail disorders** 103
    Splinter haemorrhages 103
    Fungal infections 103
    Beau's lines 105
    Clubbing 105

1 | Complications of Injury

The hand is liable to injury in many industrial, household and sporting activities. No matter what the type of injury, its severity or the structures involved, careful initial assessment and correct management are of key importance in the preservation of function and avoidance of complications.

Swelling

Swelling of the hand (Fig. 1) is caused by crushing injuries, dependency and immobility. A protein-rich fluid fills the tissue planes and, if not dispersed, will encourage a fibroblastic response causing the moving parts of the hand to adhere with disastrous loss of function. Swelling must be minimised by keeping the injured hand elevated.

Contractures

Improper splinting in an undesirable position will encourage contractures of the collateral ligaments of the small joints in the hand (Fig. 2) and may convert a minor injury into a permanent disability. Incorrect splintage must be avoided (see p. 7).

Sudeck's osteodys-trophy

Post-traumatic osteodystrophy can occur if the patient is not encouraged to use the injured hand as soon as possible. Pain, stiffness, vasomotor changes and patchy osteodystrophy (Fig. 3) are the features of this condition which is difficult to treat, but relatively easy to prevent. Careful supervision by an experienced surgeon, skilled physiotherapy and appropriate rehabilitation must be available to all patients with hand injuries, no matter how trivial the injury may appear.

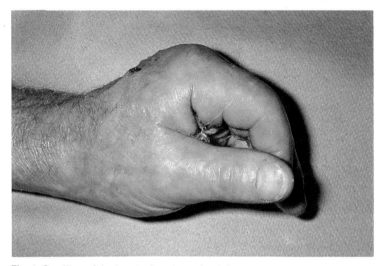

Fig. 1 Swelling of the hand a few days after injury.

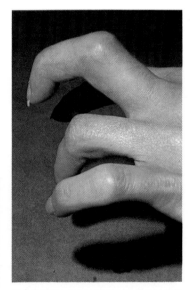

Fig. 2 This deformity was the result of treating an undisplaced fracture of the finger in a flexed position (p. 7).

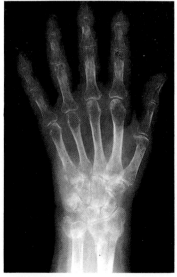

Fig. 3 Sudeck's osteodystrophy, secondary to an undisplaced fracture of the distal radius.

Elevation and Splintage

Swelling of the hand will diminish considerably after a few hours of elevation.

Dangers of sling

The traditional broad arm sling is useless and often dangerous in hand injuries for it may allow the hand to adopt a dependent position and cause constriction of the wrist at the edge of the sling.

Correct elevation

If the hand is swollen it should be elevated in a roller towel (Fig. 4). This will require a hospital admission but will almost certainly prevent a much longer subsequent admission and prolonged period of out-patient treatment.

Position of splintage

If the hand must be splinted for any length of time it is important to keep the ligamentous structures of the joints of the digits at their full length to prevent contractures. The ligaments are fully stretched when the interphalangeal joints are straight and the metacarpophalangeal joints flexed to 90° or, in the case of the thumb, when it is fully abducted from the palm (Fig. 5).

Boxing glove

This position can be maintained by a boxing glove dressing (Fig. 6) in which the fingers are splinted around a pad of fluffed gauze in the palm by wool and crepe bandages. The wrist must be kept dorsiflexed and this is best done by reinforcing the boxing glove dressing with a plaster back slab.

Volar slab

As an alternative to the boxing glove dressing the hand may be placed in a volar slab in the position shown in Fig. 5.

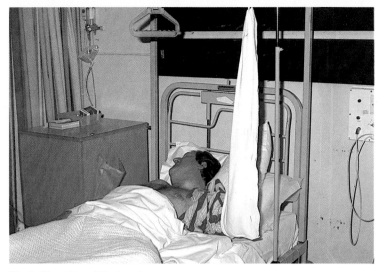

Fig. 4 Elevation of the hand.

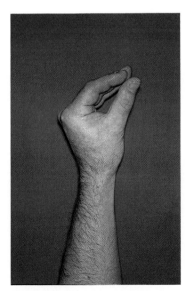

Fig. 5 The correct position for immobilisation.

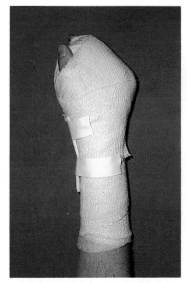

Fig. 6 A boxing glove dressing.

Undisplaced

Undisplaced fractures of the phalanges with a stable configuration (Fig. 7) do not need elaborate treatment. Healing is rapid and movement of the finger should be encouraged as soon as pain and swelling allow.

Displaced

Displaced fractures (Fig. 8) should be reduced and held in the corrected position on a splint for 2−3 weeks. When the fracture is clinically stable, supervised mobilisation is allowed.

If the fracture is unstable and redisplacement occurs, then internal fixation may be necessary, although the majority of phalangeal fractures can be managed by conservative methods. The degree of displacement should be assessed from radiographs of good quality taken in two planes at right angles to each other. Further films are taken during the period of splintage to check if redisplacement has occurred. Union is confirmed by checking the stability of the fracture on clinical examination, not by radiological examination, because the fracture line remains visible for a long period.

Condyles

Fractures of the condyles of the phalanges are often difficult to control (Fig. 9) and internal fixation with a fine Kirschner wire may be preferable to external splintage. Malunited fractures, especially of the proximal phalanx, produce an unsightly deformity of the finger (Fig. 10).

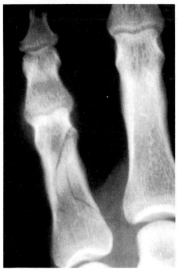

Fig. 7 A stable undisplaced fracture of the proximal phalanx.

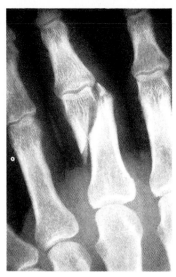

Fig. 8 An unstable displaced fracture of the proximal phalanx.

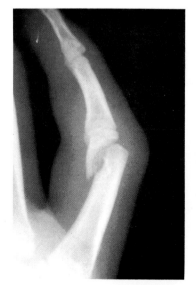

Fig. 9 A fracture of a phalangeal condyle.

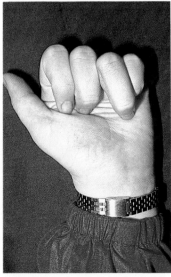

Fig. 10 Malunion of a fracture of the proximal phalanx of the finger.

Fractures of the Phalanges (2)

Garter strapping

Stable fractures may be treated by splinting the injured finger to an adjacent one (Fig. 11). It is important to place cotton wool between the fingers to prevent pressure sores and the strapping should leave the joints free to move.

Splintage

Most phalangeal fractures can be treated on a metal splint padded with foam rubber (Fig. 12). If correctly applied this will hold most fractures in position after reduction. The 90° bend in the splint should correspond to the metacarpophalangeal joint, the surface marking of which is the distal palmar skin crease. To avoid malrotation, the palmar part of the splint should point to the tuberosity of the scaphoid; the fingertips converge on this point in flexion. Malrotation of the fingers can be identified by looking at the fingernails from the tips of the fingers. Normally the nails of all four fingers make a smooth arc which is broken when one is out of alignment.

Dangerous splintage

Strapping the fingers straight on a tongue spatula (Fig. 13) or flexed over a roller bandage (Fig. 14) should be totally forbidden because these methods do not respect the correct position for splintage of the hand and functionally disastrous contractures are likely to follow their use.

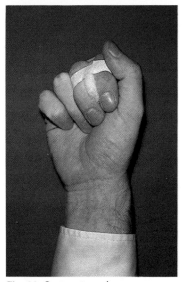

Fig. 11 Garter strapping.

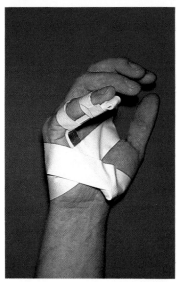

Fig. 12 The use of a padded metal splint for fractures of the fingers.

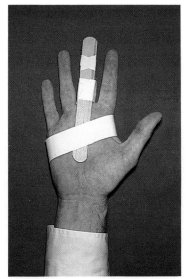

Fig. 13 Metacarpophalangeal joint splinted in extension. Incorrect.

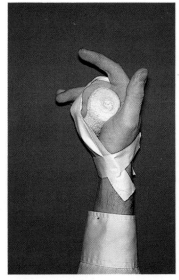

Fig. 14 Interphalangeal joints splinted in flexion. Incorrect.

4 | Fractures of Metacarpal Bones

Isolated fractures of the shafts of the metacarpal bones are usually stable and, as they are splinted by adjacent bones, additional splintage is unnecessary. Displaced fractures may need reduction and stabilisation. Multiple fractures are often associated with considerable swelling with its attendant risks of stiffness and contracture (p. 1).

Bennett's fracture

This is a fracture–dislocation of the base of the metacarpal bone of the thumb (Fig. 15). The small fragment remains in the correct position, held by the intermetacarpal ligament, while the whole first ray is pulled proximally by the abductor pollicis longus muscle. When the fracture is reduced and held by a cast there is a tendency for it to redisplace so it is better to hold the reduction with a Kirschner wire driven through the thumb metacarpal into the carpus or the adjacent metacarpal bone. The wire can be removed 3 or 4 weeks later.

'Boxer's fracture'

A fracture through the neck of the little finger metacarpal bone (Fig. 16) is extremely common and is caused by striking an object with the ungloved fist. Splintage is not necessary and early active mobilisation should be encouraged. Some loss of prominence of the knuckle at the base of the little finger is to be expected, but does not interfere with hand function (Fig. 17). The uncommon fracture that is associated with gross angulation of the head of the metacarpal bone, judged on a true lateral radiograph of the hand, should be reduced and stabilised with a Kirschner wire.

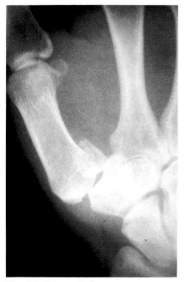

Fig. 15 Bennett's fracture.

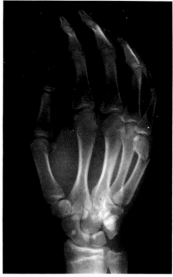

Fig. 16 'Boxer's fracture'.

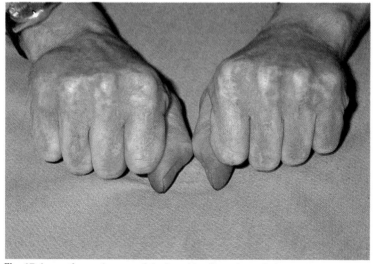

Fig. 17 Loss of prominence of the knuckle after a boxer's fracture in the right hand.

5 | Carpal Injuries

Fracture of the scaphoid

The scaphoid is usually broken in a fall on the hand. The wrist is painful and there is swelling and tenderness in the 'anatomical snuff-box' at the base of the thumb. If a fracture of the scaphoid is suspected but not confirmed on X-ray examination (Fig. 18) it is wise to place the wrist in plaster and arrange for a further examination in about 10 days. Most fractures of the scaphoid will unite after splintage for 6 weeks but delayed union sometimes occurs and bone-grafting may be necessary. Established non-unions (Fig. 19) often present when a patient complains of pain in a wrist that was 'badly sprained' some years before.

Dislocated lunate

This injury (Fig. 20) is one of a group of carpal dislocations sharing a similar mechanism of injury. Sometimes the other carpal bones are displaced and the lunate retains its position relative to the radius — a peri-lunate dislocation. Such dislocations are associated with complex ligamentous disruptions and intercarpal instability may persist after reduction.

Kienböck's disease

Avascular necrosis of the lunate (Fig. 21) is thought to be due to minor trauma. It causes pain in the wrist. There is sclerosis and collapse of the lunate and osteoarthritic changes may supervene.

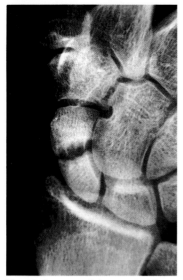

Fig. 18 Fracture of the scaphoid.

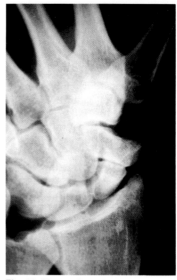

Fig. 19 Non-union of the scaphoid. Osteo-arthritic changes are present in the wrist.

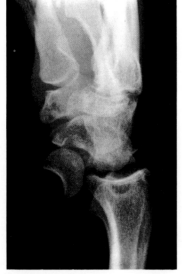

Fig. 20 Dislocation of the lunate. Lateral view.

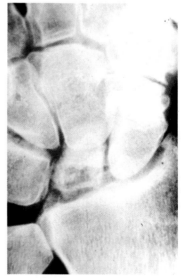

Fig. 21 Kienböck's disease.

Inter-phalangeal dislocations

The proximal interphalangeal joints are the most frequently dislocated joints in the hand. The intermediate phalanx is dislocated dorsally (Fig. 22), laterally or, rarely, anteriorly. Even though the diagnosis is usually obvious on clinical examination an X-ray examination should be ordered before and after reduction to exclude associated fractures and check congruity of reduction. Reduction is straightforward and can be carried out with ring-block anaesthesia. Damage to the collateral ligaments should be excluded by stressing them after reduction (Fig. 23); if a ligament is torn, surgical repair may be necessary. If the interphalangeal joint is stable it should be splinted in the extended position on a short metal splint for a few days.

Spindle finger

Ligamentous injuries of the proximal interphalangeal joint, whether or not the joint has been dislocated, are often followed by prolonged swelling (Fig. 24) and discomfort. Patients should be warned that this may occur as they are often reluctant to move the joint when it is swollen. Stiffness and flexion contractures can rapidly become established in the proximal interphalangeal joint after injury, but can be prevented by correct splintage and early mobilisation when discomfort allows.

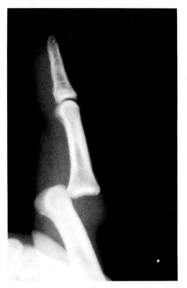

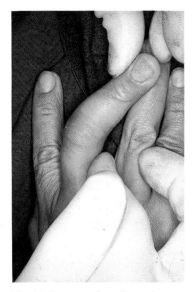

Fig. 22 Dorsal dislocation of the proximal interphalangeal joint.

Fig. 23 Rupture of a collateral ligament.

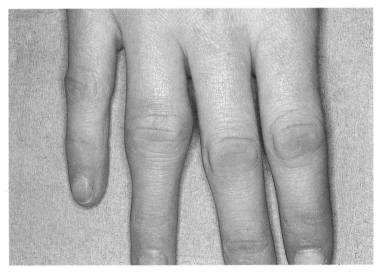

Fig. 24 Swelling of the proximal interphalangeal joint after a minor sprain.

Joint Injuries (2)

Metacarpo-phalangeal of thumb

A sprain or rupture of the ulnar collateral ligament of the metacarpophalangeal joint of the thumb are common injuries. They are caused by abduction strains applied to the thumb, often during sporting activities. Chronic stretching related to occupation may also occur ('game-keeper's thumb').

An acute sprain should be treated in a forearm plaster incorporating the thumb for 3–4 weeks. If the ligament has been completely ruptured this is not an effective form of treatment because healing is prevented by the adductor aponeurosis which becomes interposed between the ligament and the base of the proximal phalanx of the thumb. Operative repair is imperative if a chronically unstable thumb is to be avoided.

Rupture of the ligament should be confirmed by stressing the joint after injecting local anaesthetic into the tender area (Fig. 25). Radiographic examination will show a subluxation (Fig. 26) or occasionally a fragment of bone avulsed from the proximal phalanx (Fig. 27). The ulnar collateral ligament is attached to this piece of bone.

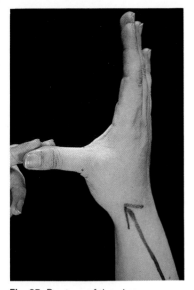

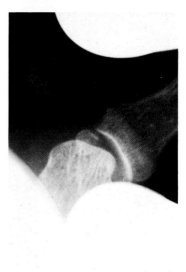

Fig. 25 Rupture of the ulnar collateral ligament of the metacarpophalangeal joint of the thumb.

Fig. 26 Subluxation shown radiographically on a stress view.

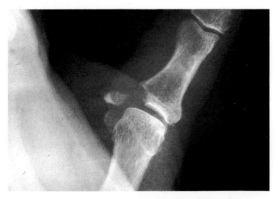

Fig. 27 A fragment of bone avulsed from the ulnar border of the proximal phalanx indicates an unstable injury. Note the rotation of the fragment.

Flexor tendons

Division of a flexor tendon in the hand is a serious injury that is often associated with some permanent disability. Such an injury is usually caused by a sharp object, for example, gripping a knife blade, falling on broken glass or when opening a tin. The site of the injury should make the examiner suspicious that a tendon may be damaged.

Diagnosis is not usually difficult. When the hand is relaxed in a supinated position with the wrist extended the fingers make a 'cascade' with the degree of flexion increasing from index to little finger (Fig. 28). This posture is determined by the resting tone in the muscles and is altered when the deep flexor tendon or both tendons to the finger are cut (Fig. 29) but not when the superficialis tendon alone is cut. The actions of the tendons should also be tested and sensation and circulation in the fingers should also be checked because digital nerves and vessels may have been injured. Primary repair of flexor tendons should only be done by an expert. Injuries between the distal palmar skin crease and the middle of the finger ('No Man's Land') where the tendons lie in the fibrous flexor sheath are particularly difficult to deal with as adhesions invariably form and unless special techniques are used the excursion of the tendons will be limited. For this reason delayed flexor tendon grafting is preferred by some surgeons.

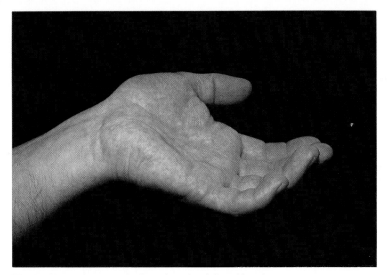

Fig. 28 Normal posture in the relaxed uninjured hand.

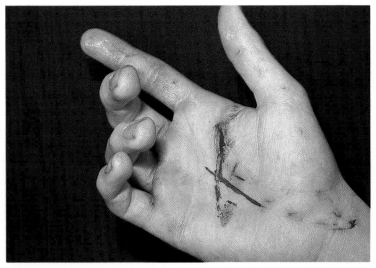

Fig. 29 The superficial and deep flexor tendons of the index finger have been cut in the palm.

Avulsion of flexor tendon

The ring finger is almost invariably affected. It can readily be confirmed on one's own hand that the metacarpophalangeal joint of the ring finger has limited extension when the other fingers are flexed in the palm. The injury often happens when a rugby player grasps the shirt of another player and the ring finger is forcibly extended whilst the other fingers remain in the gripping position. The deep flexor tendon is avulsed from the terminal phalanx and may retract into the palm. The patient is unable to flex the terminal interphalangeal joint (Fig. 30). Early surgical repair is indicated and the results are usually good.

Extensor tendon injury

The long extensors on the wrist and back of the hand are usually damaged in sharp cutting injuries. The patient is unable to extend the affected fingers at the metacarpophalangeal joint (Fig. 31). Extension of the interphalangeal joints is still possible because this is performed by the intrinsic muscles acting on the intact extensor expansion of the fingers.

Primary tendon repair has a much better prognosis than in flexor tendon injuries, but careful supervision following operation is still necessary if a good result is to be obtained. Tendon grafting or tendon transfer may be necessary in the late case.

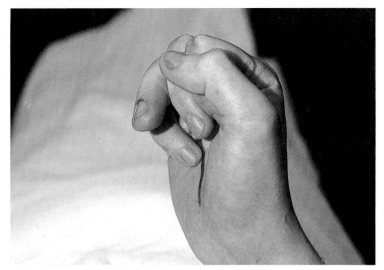

Fig. 30 Avulsion of the deep flexor tendon of the ring finger. Patient attempting to make a fist.

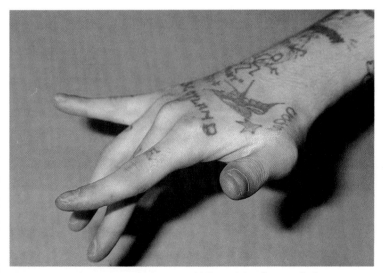

Fig. 31 Cut long extensor tendons to middle and ring fingers. Patient attempting to extend all fingers.

Mallet finger

A rupture of the extensor mechanism at its insertion into the terminal phalanx, often caused by a trivial flexion injury. The distal phalanx cannot be actively extended and lies in about 20–60° of flexion (Fig. 32). The injury is treated by keeping the distal interphalangeal joint extended in a simple plastic splint for about 6 weeks.

Boutonniere deformity

This deformity occurs when the central slip of the extensor expansion is cut or ruptured on the dorsum of the proximal interphalangeal joint. The lateral bands of the extensor apparatus slip laterally and anteriorly, eventually acting as flexors of the proximal interphalangeal joint and hyper-extending the distal interphalangeal joint (Fig. 33). The injury should be recognised early and treated by splintage or operative repair because correction of the established deformity is difficult and not always successful.

Extensor pollicis longus tendon

This tendon may rupture spontaneously after a Colles' fracture or when the wrist is affected by rheumatoid arthritis (Fig. 34). The patient may feel something snap and is unable to extend the interphalangeal joint of the thumb. This action can be restored by transferring the tendon of extensor indicis proprius to the distal part of the ruptured tendon.

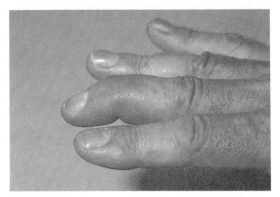
Fig. 32 Mallet finger.

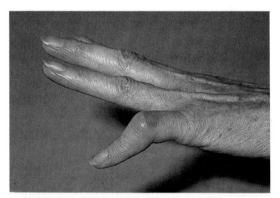
Fig. 33 Boutonnière deformity.

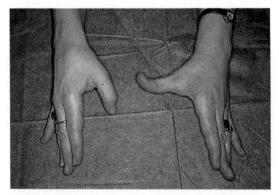
Fig. 34 Rupture of the tendon of extensor pollicis longus in the right hand.

8 | Nerve Injuries (1)

The hand is supplied by the median and ulnar nerves, which contain both sensory and motor fibres, and the radial nerve which supplies sensation to the radial border of the back of the hand. Nerves may be damaged in any open injury of the hand. Nerve repair should be carried out by an expert; full recovery is not always achieved in mixed nerves in adults but useful functional recovery is gained in many cases.

Median nerve

The median nerve in the hand supplies the abductor pollicis brevis, the opponens pollicis, the radial two lumbricals and may give a motor supply to the flexor pollicis brevis muscle. It gives sensation to the skin over the thenar eminence, the palmar aspect of the thumb and the radial two and a half fingers. Variations in the motor and sensory supply are not uncommon and there is also overlap with adjacent sensory areas.

When the median nerve is divided the patient is unable to abduct the thumb (Fig. 35). Wasting of the median innervated muscles will follow (Fig. 36).

Damage to the median nerve is very serious because the thumb cannot be positioned against the fingers and sensation is lost in the 'picking-up' area of the hand.

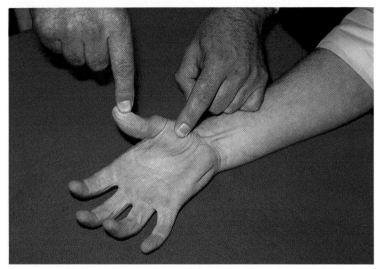

Fig. 35 Testing normal abduction of the thumb against resistance. Contraction of the muscles is visible and palpable.

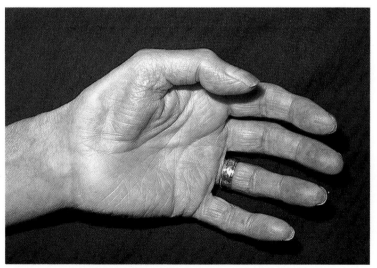

Fig. 36 Visible wasting of the abductor pollicis brevis muscle.

8 | Nerve Injuries (2)

Ulnar nerve

The ulnar nerve supplies those intrinsic muscles of the hand not supplied by the median nerve. It supplies sensation to the palmar aspect of the ulnar one and a half digits and the whole of the back of the hand, except for the area supplied by the radial nerve. Division of the ulnar nerve at the wrist is followed by wasting of intrinsic muscles most obviously the first dorsal interosseous, and the little and ring fingers adopt a position of slight flexion — the 'ulnar claw hand' (Fig. 37).

When the patient attempts to grip a flat object between the thumb and the hand, the flexor pollicis longus (innervated by the median nerve) comes into action causing flexion at the interphalangeal joint — Froment's sign (Fig. 38). The patient is unable to grip a piece of paper between two fingers because the interossei are paralysed (Fig. 39); the hand must be kept flat when carrying out this test to avoid trick movements using the extrinsic muscles.

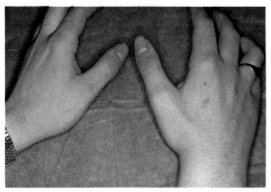

Fig. 37 Wasting of the first dorsal interosseous muscle and slight clawing of the ulnar two fingers of the right hand.

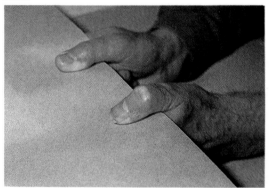

Fig. 38 Positive Froment's sign in the left hand.

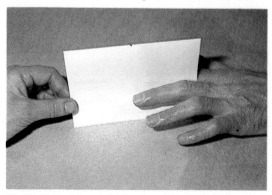

Fig. 39 Patient (on right) is attempting to hold the sheet of paper against a gentle pull from the examiner.

9 | Finger Tip Injuries (1)

An apparently minor injury of the fingertip can be followed by marked disability unless treatment is carefully supervised. The aim is to achieve early sound healing so that the patient may use the finger in normal activities.

Subungual haematoma

Crushing injuries of the fingertip, for example, catching a finger in the door of a car, can cause painful extravasation of blood beneath the nail (Fig. 40). There may be an associated fracture of the terminal phalanx, but this can usually be ignored because it is well splinted by the nail. In the acute phase the blood should be drained from beneath the nail by drilling a couple of holes through the nail with a fine wire, such as a straightened paper clip, which has been heated with a match until it is red hot.

Nail dislocation

A more serious injury occurs when the nail is dislocated from its bed (Fig. 41). This is often associated with a displaced fracture of the terminal phalanx which is usually an open fracture (Fig. 42). The nail should not be removed but returned to its bed so that it may stabilise the fracture and prevent adhesions forming between the layers of the nail fold. A short splint should be taped to the finger for 2 weeks.

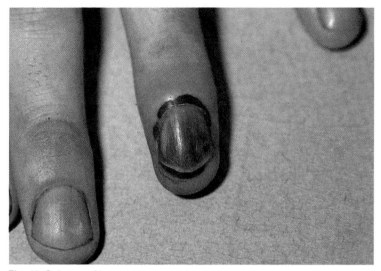

Fig. 40 Subungual haematoma.

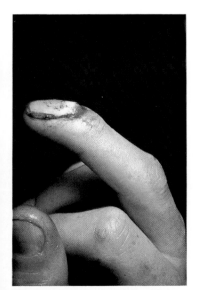

Fig. 41 Displacement of the nail from the nail fold.

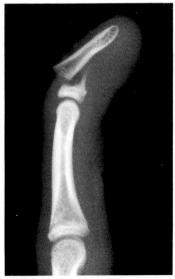

Fig. 42 The associated fracture of the terminal phalanx.

9 | Finger Tip Injuries (2)

Partial amputations

Partial amputations are common industrial injuries (Fig. 43). The aim of treatment is to restore a pain-free finger tip with sensation and stable skin cover.

The wound can frequently be closed primarily if the terminal phalanx is trimmed. Alternatively the skin can be replaced using small local skin flaps. Small areas of skin loss without exposure of the bone can be allowed to heal secondarily.

If most of the distal phalanx has been lost there is no support for the nail and it may grow in a curled and unsightly way (Fig. 44). Ablation of the nail may be necessary.

Small remnants of the nail bed will continue to produce nail tissue and this may form a mass of keratin (Fig. 45) or a spike of nail. The remains of the germinal matrix of the nail should be removed.

HAND CONDITIONS

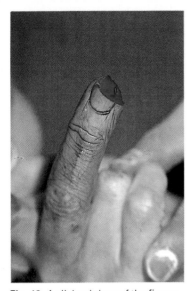

Fig. 43 A slicing injury of the finger tip.

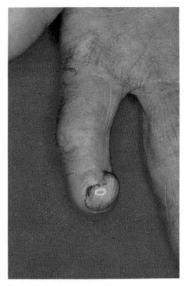

Fig. 44 Deformed nail growth following a partial amputation of the tip of the finger.

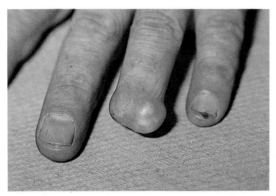

Fig. 45 A keratin-filled lesion caused by continued growth of nail remnants.

| # Special Types of Injury (1)

**Major crush
injuries**

Major crushing injuries (Fig. 46) are often due to
industrial accidents involving machinery such as
presses. Initial treatment consists of removal of
all dead tissue and tissue of doubtful viability, and
obtaining skin cover, which may involve pedicled
skin grafts. Further reconstructive procedures
must be planned for each patient, the aim being
to provide a hand with sensation that is capable of
gripping.

**Wringer
injuries**

Wringer or roller injuries cause crushing of all
tissues in the hand and the skin may be stripped
off underlying structures. Distally based flaps
(Fig. 47) are seldom viable and should not be
stitched back into place. Skin replacement, using
the techniques of plastic surgery, should be
carried out as soon as possible.

**Guillotine
injuries**

Clean cut amputations (Fig. 48) and those with
minimal crushing are suitable for replantation
using microsurgical techniques. The amputated
part should be sealed in a sterile plastic bag,
placed on ice and sent with the patient without
delay to a centre with microsurgical facilities.

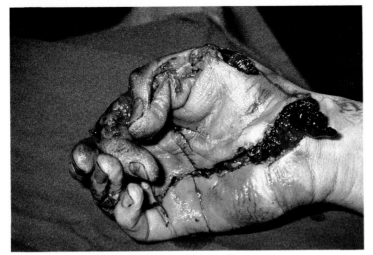

Fig. 46 Crushing injury caused by a book-binding press.

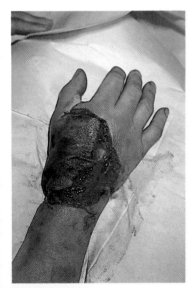

Fig. 47 Roller injury. Note that the distally based skin flap is clearly dead.

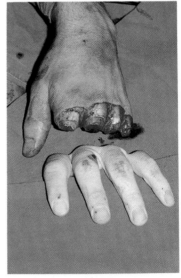

Fig. 48 Industrial guillotine injury.

Special Types of Injury (2)

Injection injuries

Injuries caused by high pressure injection guns may appear trivial (Fig. 49) but foreign material such as grease is forced into the tissues and extensive tissue necrosis will occur unless the material is removed promptly. An early and wide exploration of the hand is necessary.

Burns

Burns vary from the superficial to the extensive deep burn. A special category is the electrical burn, which is nearly always much deeper than it appears. The cornerstones of treatment are control of oedema, maintenance of movement and relief of pain. Excision of dead tissue and replacement by skin grafts will be necessary in deep burns (Fig. 50). Further surgery may be needed to restore movement by tendon grafts or to release contractures. Expert rehabilitation is essential.

Frostbite

Cold injury causes necrosis of finger tips (Fig. 51). In the acute phase the whole patient should be warmed and low molecular weight dextran given intravenously. The role of sympathectomy is not established. Amputation should be delayed until there is a clear line of demarcation between living and dead tissue.

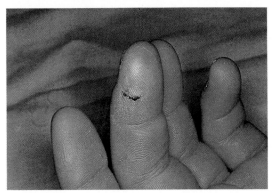

Fig. 49 High pressure greasegun injury. Adequate early exploration and decompression must be performed.

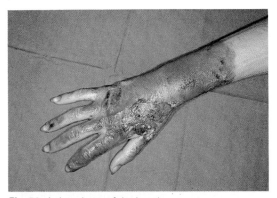

Fig. 50 A deep burn of the hand.

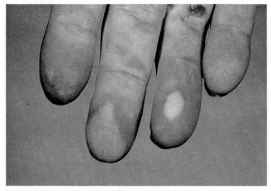

Fig. 51 Frostbite of the fingertips.

11 | Self-inflicted Injuries

Slashed wrist

'Wrist-slashing' is common. It may be an attention-seeking gesture or a seriously intended attempt at suicide. All patients should be assessed by a psychiatrist. Typically there are several cuts which may vary in depth (Fig. 52). Considerable damage may be caused to deeper structures even when this was not intended. These patients are often unco-operative when the hand is examined; if there is any doubt about the extent of damage the wrist should be explored when the patient's condition allows and divided structures repaired. As might be expected, these patients pose a difficult problem of rehabilitation and the wrist-slashing may be repeated.

Dermatitis artefacta

The possibility of self-inflicted injury should be thought of when a patient has odd skin lesions that show no specific abnormality on biopsy but which refuse to heal despite various forms of treatment. Dermatitis artefacta takes many forms such as repeated scratching with some object (Fig. 53) or multiple cigarette burns. The lesions tend to heal if the area is kept occluded, for example, with a plaster cast, but the cast may be removed by the patient for a seemingly plausible reason. Even when it is obvious that the lesion is self-inflicted this may be blandly denied by the patient but a skilled psychiatrist is often able to elicit a reason for this type of behaviour.

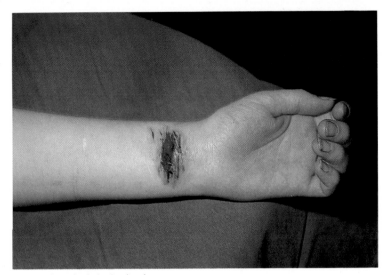

Fig. 52 A typical slashed wrist.

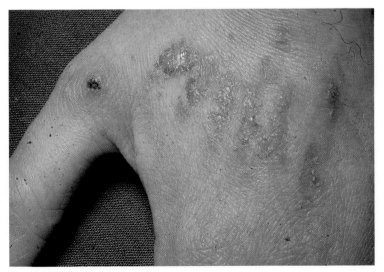

Fig. 53 Dermatitis artefacta.

Amputation of a finger may be required for severe injury, infection, malignant disease or severe deformity, for example due to Dupuytren's contracture.

Index finger

If the amputation produces significant shortening, the stump of the index finger is of little use and the patient tends to bypass it when using a pinch grip (Fig. 54).

Amputation through the metacarpophalangeal joint leaves an unsightly projection caused by the metacarpal head; an oblique amputation through the metacarpal gives a better cosmetic result (Fig. 55).

Middle and ring fingers

The ideal level of amputation is debatable. The finger is often removed at the metacarpo-phalangeal joint but many surgeons prefer to leave a small stump of the proximal phalanx to prevent objects slipping between the fingers (Fig. 56). An alternative is to remove the finger and its metacarpal (ray amputation).

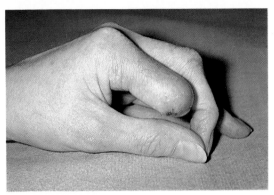

Fig. 54 A short stump of the index finger is not used when gripping small objects.

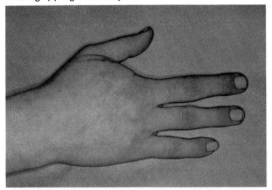

Fig. 55 The appearance of the hand of another patient after amputation of the index finger through the metacarpal bone.

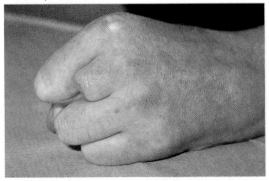

Fig. 56 A small stump of the middle or ring fingers prevents objects slipping from the palm.

12 | **Finger Amputations (2)**

Little finger

The little and ring fingers are important for stabilising objects gripped strongly by the hand. A weak power grip results when these fingers are lost by amputation (Fig. 57) or cannot be brought into the palm because of stiffness. When there is only a short stump of the little finger this adds little to grip strength, and the cosmetic appearance of the hand can be improved by amputation through the metacarpal, which gives a smooth contour to the ulnar border of the hand.

Thumb

The ability to oppose the thumb to the fingers is of supreme importance in the function of the hand. Every effort should be made to preserve functional length of the thumb in partial amputations, although tightly stretched, unstable skin over the stump should be avoided.

Complete loss of the thumb (Fig. 58) is a major injury and the hand can function only as a paddle or hook. Microsurgical replantation of a traumatically amputated thumb should be considered if the circumstances are favourable (Fig. 59). If this is not possible secondary procedures to construct a new thumb will be necessary. Several procedures have been devised including the transfer of a toe to the hand, construction of a thumb from the index finger (pollicisation) and lengthening the thumb metacarpal to provide an opposition post.

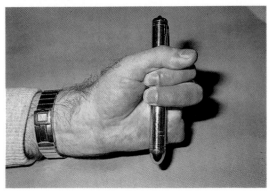

Fig. 57 An unstable power grip when the little and ring fingers have been lost.

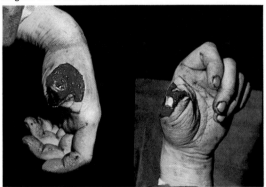

Fig. 58 Complete amputation of the thumb in an accident.

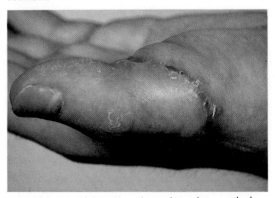

Fig. 59 Successful replantation using microsurgical techniques.

13 | Congenital Anomalies (1)

Classification

Failure of formation   Constriction bands
Failure of separation Miscellaneous
Duplication   Associated with
Overgrowth   generalised skeletal
                          abnormalities.
Examples of each will be illustrated.

Aetiology

The anomalies may affect the hand only or be part of a malformation syndrome or skeletal dysplasia. There may be a clear pattern of inheritance or the deformity may be sporadic (e.g. thalidomide deformities).

Treatment

May not be necessary; it should be directed to improving function rather than cosmesis. Major reconstructive procedures should be completed before school age if possible.

Failure of formation

Transverse

The commonest site is the upper third of the forearm (Fig. 60). The deformity is not inherited and treatment is by early prosthetic fitting.

   Distal transverse defects in the hand (Fig. 61) are sporadic in occurrence. They may be amenable to surgical reconstruction, e.g. by transferring a toe to the hand by microvascular techniques.

Longitudinal

Distal radial deficiency or radial club hand (Fig. 62) is sporadic in occurrence but was a common deformity caused by thalidomide. Treatment is directed towards providing a useful hand in a functional position; this involves centralising the hand on the ulna and constructing a thumb using one of the fingers (pollicisation). If the elbow is very stiff elaborate reconstruction is not indicated as the child will be unable to reach the mouth with the hand.

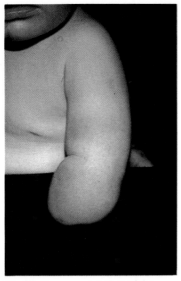

Fig. 60 Transverse deficit of the forearm.

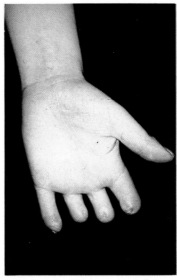

Fig. 61 A distal transverse deficit.

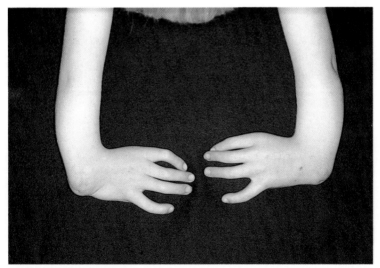

Fig. 62 Radial club hands.

Congenital Anomalies (2)

Failure of separation

Syndactyly

Syndactyly (incomplete separation of the digits) is the most common type. Syndactyly may be an isolated abnormality or associated with a generalised disorder. The inheritance is variable.

Simple syndactyly

In simple syndactyly (Fig. 63) the fingers are joined by skin alone. They can be separated by relatively simple plastic surgical procedures with a reasonable expectation of a good cosmetic and functional result.

Complex syndactyly

A syndactyly is complex if both skin and bone are joined. Acrosyndactyly is a deformity in which the fingers are joined distally often leaving a space between the fingers more proximally. In Apert's syndrome (Fig. 64) complex bilateral syndactyly is associated with characteristic craniofacial abnormalities. Surgical treatment of complex syndactyly is difficult, but worthwhile.

Duplication

Polydactyly

Polydactyly (Fig. 65), the possession of extra digits, is fairly common. It may be an isolated hand abnormality, when it can be transmitted by autosomal dominant inheritance, or part of a generalised congenital disorder in which case transmission may be by an autosomal recessive mode (Fig. 77). An obviously abnormal and functionless digit can be removed.

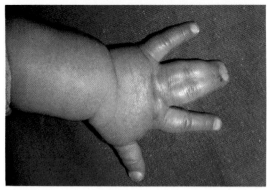

Fig. 63 Simple syndactyly.

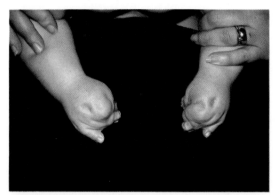

Fig. 64 Complex syndactyly in Apert's syndrome.

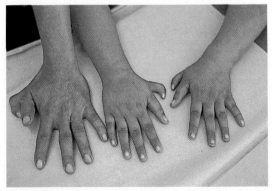

Fig. 65 Bilateral pre-axial polydactyly. The other hand belongs to the patient's father.

Overgrowth

Macrodactyly

Macrodactyly is localised gigantism of a digit. Primary macrodactyly (Fig. 66) is usually unilateral and one or more fingers are involved. It usually occurs within the first 2 years of life. All tissues in the fingers are affected; the subcutaneous fat is hypertrophic and the digital nerves are thickened.

Treatment is difficult. An attempt can be made to improve the appearance by local tissue resection but this is not always satisfactory and amputation may be necessary if the appearance is very bizarre and the finger has no function.

Neurofibro-matosis

A similar condition of the fingers may occur in neurofibromatosis (Fig. 67) but in this condition there is also abnormal pigmentation of the skin and often other skeletal abnormalities and soft tissue tumours. The condition is transmitted by autosomal dominant inheritance.

Constriction bands

Annular grooves lie at right angles to the long axis of the limb and may or may not be completely circumferential. Their occurrence is spasmodic and their cause not established. The clinical picture ranges from an intra-uterine amputation (Fig. 68) to a small groove on a finger; acrosyndactyly (p. 43) is common.

Tight constriction bands should be resected and acrosyndactyly will require separation.

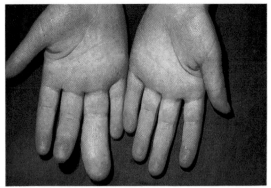

Fig. 66 Primary macrodactyly.

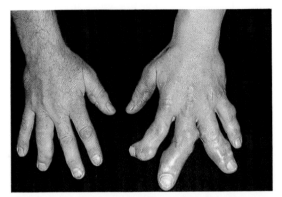

Fig. 67 Neurofibromatosis affecting both hands.

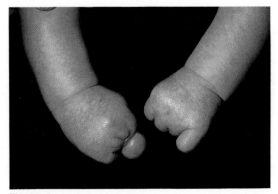

Fig. 68 Constriction bands.

Miscellaneous

**Campto-
dactyly**

A congenital flexion contracture of the proximal interphalangeal joint, most commonly affecting the little finger (Fig. 69). Often of autosomal dominant inheritance, but may be sporadic. In mild cases function is good and treatment is unnecessary. Severe deformities cannot be corrected by splintage and surgery may be required.

**Triphalangeal
thumb**

The thumb contains an extra phalanx and the digit may have the appearance and movements of a finger — the 'five-fingered hand' (Fig. 70). As the radial digit cannot be opposed to the other fingers surgical treatment is necessary to place it in a position where it may be used as a thumb.

**Arthrogry-
phosis**

Children with this sporadic disorder are born with stiff limbs and deformities of the hands (Fig. 71) and feet. The cause is unknown; the limb muscles are poorly developed, but this may be secondary to an underlying neurological disorder. Treatment of the hand deformities is seldom, if ever, necessary because the function is often surprisingly good and any disability may be related more to stiffness in the elbow and shoulder.

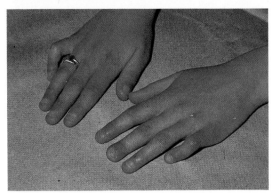

Fig. 69 Camptodactyly.

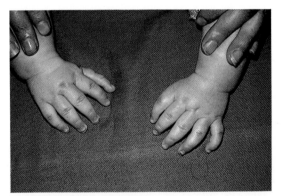

Fig. 70 Five-fingered hands.

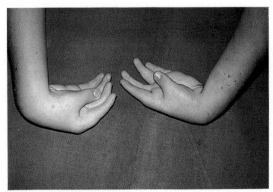

Fig. 71 Arthrogryphosis.

Generalised skeletal abnormalities

In these disorders the hand abnormality is a manifestation of a condition affecting other parts of the skeleton.

Ollier's disease (multiple enchondromatosis)

An uncommon disorder of sporadic occurrence in which cartilaginous masses develop on several bones. The condition may be bilateral but is not symmetrical in distribution. Sometimes the masses are so large that amputation is necessary (Fig. 72). Malignant change is a complication. Mafucci's syndrome is Ollier's disease associated with multiple haemangiomata.

Marfan's syndrome

A generalised connective tissue disorder inherited by autosomal dominant transmission. The patients are taller than normal and have long slender hands (Fig. 73) and feet, hence the alternative name of arachnodactyly. Camptodactyly (p. 47) and clinodactyly (excessive lateral curvature of the fingers) are frequently associated. Other features of the disorder may include scoliosis, dislocation of the lenses of the eye, aortic aneurysm and aortic incompetence.

Achondroplasia

A relatively common condition of autosomal dominant inheritance. Patients have short limbs but the head and trunk are of relatively normal proportion. The hand tends to be short and stubby (Fig. 74) and the fingers are held in an abducted position — the 'trident hand'.

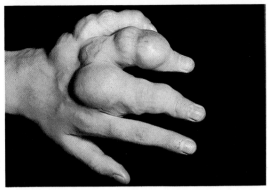

Fig. 72 Ollier's disease. A particularly severe example.

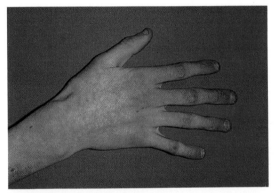

Fig. 73 Marfan's syndrome.

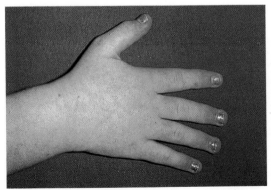

Fig. 74 Achondroplasia.

Congenital Anomalies (6)

Generalised skeletal abnormalities (co)

Morquio's syndrome

One of several disorders of mucopolysaccharide metabolism, Morquio's syndrome has an autosomal recessive type of inheritance, as is usual with inborn errors of metabolism. The condition becomes apparent between the ages of 1 and 3 years of age with dwarfing, coarsening of facial features, hepatomegaly, a flared rib cage and bulging sternum. The hands are short and stubby (Fig. 75).

Nail–patella syndrome

Synonym: onycho-osteodysplasia.
A condition of autosomal dominant inheritance, in which there is hypoplasia and splitting of the nails, most commonly those of the thumb (Fig. 76), associated with hypoplasia or absence of the patellae, bony abnormalities of the elbows and a curious bony spur on the ilium which is often palpable.

Ellis – Van Crefeld syndrome

Synonym: chondroectodermal dysplasia.
A dysplasia of autosomal recessive inheritance. Clinical features include short stature, postaxial polydactyly (Fig. 77), nail hypoplasia and cardiac defects in half those affected. Teeth may be present in the neonate with this disorder.

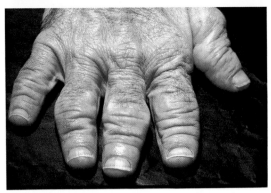

Fig. 75 Morquio's syndrome.

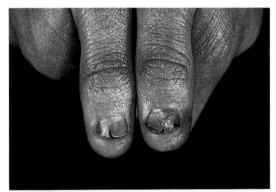

Fig. 76 Nail–patella syndrome.

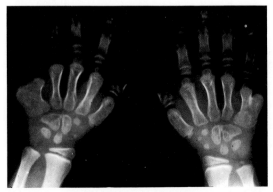

Fig. 77 Postaxial polydactyly in the Ellis – Van Crefeld syndrome.

Hand Infections (1)

The classic bacterial hand infections described in many textbooks are now seldom seen, perhaps because of early treatment with antibiotics; nevertheless, infections can still severely damage the hand unless treated early and well. The essentials of treatment are splintage and elevation of the hand, adequate drainage of localised pus and appropriate antibiotic therapy. Staphylococci are the organisms most commonly isolated.

Pulp space

Pulp space infections (Fig. 78) often follow minor injuries.

Clinical features

The finger tip is swollen and tender and the patient suffers from a throbbing pain that prevents sleep.

Treatment

If the infection does not settle rapidly with antibiotic therapy, surgical drainage should be performed before there is damage to skin or bone.

Paronychia

Infection of the nail fold (Fig. 79) is one of the more common hand infections.

Clinical features

Redness, swelling and pain localised to the base of the nail. The infection may track completely round the nail.

Treatment

Localised pus should be released from beneath the nail by removing a corner of the nail at the germinal fold.

HAND CONDITIONS

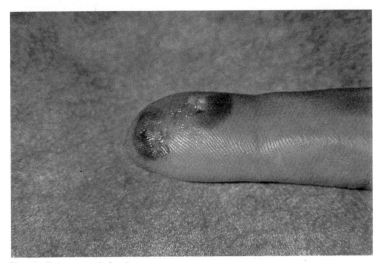

Fig. 78 Pulp space infection.

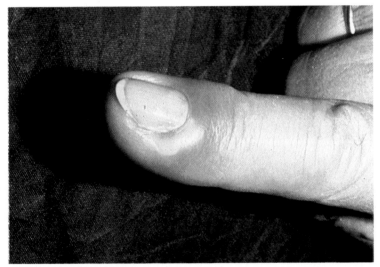

Fig. 79 Acute paronychia.

Web space

Infection in the loose tissue between the fingers may follow minor skin trauma.

Clinical features

The infection is usually well localised between the fingers. There is marked swelling, pain and pus is often pointing (Fig. 80).

Treatment

The pus should be adequately drained without delay and an appropriate antibiotic started.

Tendon sheath

Infection of the flexor tendon sheath may follow a pricking injury, but often no injury is recalled. Bites can cause particularly severe infections of the tendon sheath.

Clinical features

The finger is slightly swollen and erythematous (Fig. 81). The patient cannot move it because of pain which is aggravated by attempts at passive movement. Tenderness is localised over the line of the fibrous flexor sheath.

Treatment

Early antibiotic treatment may mask the severity of the infection and if the ability to move the finger does not return rapidly the tendon sheath should be surgically drained and irrigated. Delay in surgical treatment may result in necrosis of the tendon and a stiff, useless finger.

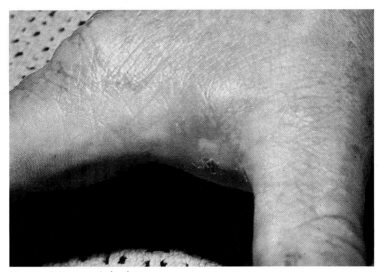

Fig. 80 Web space infection.

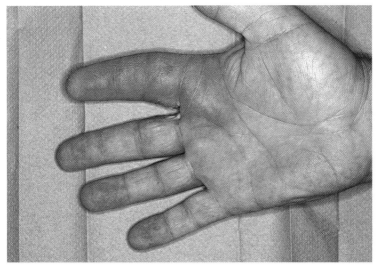

Fig. 81 Tendon sheath infection.

Septic arthritis

Usually follows a fist fight. When the knuckles strike the teeth of an opponent, organisms from the mouth can be injected into a metacarpophalangeal joint. As the hand relaxes the extensor tendon expansion seals the joint, which makes a highly effective culture chamber.

Clinical features

The patient usually seeks treatment a few days after sustaining the injury. There is severe pain, inability to move the finger and on examination a puncture wound or cut may be found over a knuckle, surrounded by cellulitis (Fig. 82).

Treatment

Early exploration and drainage of the joint is indicated before the infection causes destruction of the articular surface.

Pyogenic granuloma

An infected granuloma that follows a trivial injury. Much of the granulation tissue is beneath the skin and may be associated with a foreign body.

Clinical features

A painful red lump on the palmar surface of the hand that bleeds readily (Fig. 83).

Treatment

Excision.

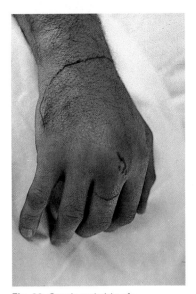

Fig. 82 Septic arthritis of a
metacarpophalangeal joint.

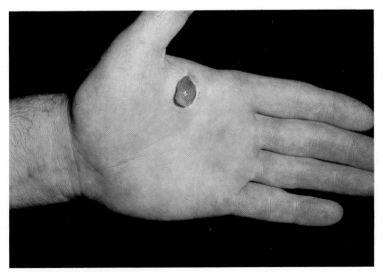

Fig. 83 Pyogenic granuloma.

Warts

The hand is a frequent site for the common wart or *verruca vulgaris* (Fig. 84). They may be isolated or multiple and are caused by a papova DNA virus.

Treatment

Many clear spontaneously; if they do not and are troublesome they can be removed by curettage or cryotherapy using liquid nitrogen.

Orf

A virus disease of sheep and goats.

Clinical features

Lesions are seen most commonly on the hand or forearm. Initially papular, they become vesicular and later pustular (Fig. 85). They are not accompanied by a systemic illness. The infection occurs in people handling the carcasses of infected animals.

Treatment

Not usually necessary as this is a self-limiting condition resolving in a few weeks.

Herpetic whitlow

Infection with Type I herpes simplex virus.

Clinical features

An extremely painful vesicular lesion on a digit (Fig. 86). It is caused by implantation of the virus in the skin through an abrasion and occurs in those who come in contact with secretions from infected persons. Dentists, nurses and medical staff are particularly at risk. Painful recurrence is common.

Treatment

Local antiviral agents such as idoxuridine may shorten the attack but do not prevent recurrence.

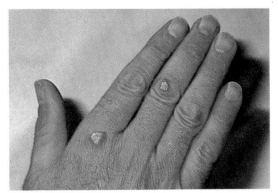

Fig. 84 Common wart.

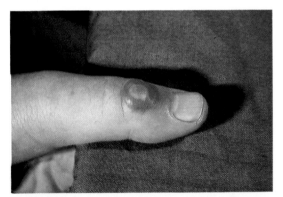

Fig. 85 Orf.

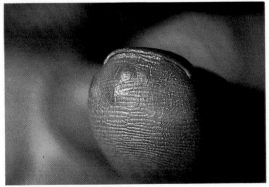

Fig. 86 Herpetic whitlow.

Erysipeloid

Infection with *Erysipelothrix insidiosa*.

Clinical features

A slowly spreading cellulitis affecting one finger (Fig. 87), or sometimes adjacent fingers without significant pain or constitutional symptoms. The infected area is a rather dull red in colour and has a raised margin at the junction with normal skin.

Erysipeloid occurs in those who handle raw meat and fish and may follow a scratch from a bone.

Treatment

The infection tends to resolve slowly without treatment, but recovery may be hastened by a short course of penicillin or tetracycline.

Scabies

Infection with *Sarcoptes scabiei hominis*, a burrowing mite. It is common and spread by close contact.

Clinical features

The hands and wrists are commonly affected. The patient complains of itching when warm, e.g. in bed at night. The typical lesion is the burrow of the mite which can be seen with a hand lens. There may be secondary changes due to scratching (Fig. 88).

Treatment

Patients and their close contacts should be treated with gamma benzene hexachloride cream or benzyl benzoate which should be applied to the whole body below the neck.

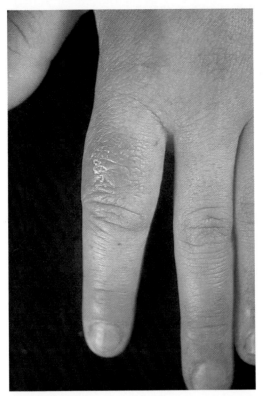

Fig. 87 Erysipeloid.

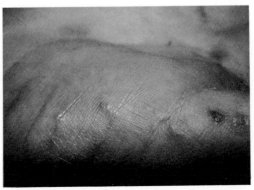

Fig. 88 Scabies.

| # Hand Infections (6)

Anthrax

Infection with *Bacillus anthracis*, a virulent sporing organism.

Clinical features

Infection can occur in those who handle the products of infected animals, such as wool, hides and bone meal. Pulmonary disease due to inhaled spores may be rapidly fatal. Local infection can be introduced by an abrasion and the hand is a common site. A pustule forms, surrounded by deep erythema and oedema and associated with regional lymphadenopathy. Bullae and vesicles form later (Fig. 89) and the organism can be isolated from them.

Treatment

Penicillin or tetracycline in high doses.

Leprosy (Hansen's disease)

A chronic infective disease due to *Mycobacterium leprae*, most prevalent in tropical and subtropical regions.

Clinical features

Manifestations are variable and depend on host–organism interactions. Skin lesions, such as hypopigmentation, and involvement of the peripheral nerves are common. The median and ulnar nerves are frequently involved and hand disability results from anaesthesia and paralysis of the intrinsic muscles (Fig. 90). The anaesthetic fingers may be lost because of secondary bacterial infection.

Treatment

The patient should be taught to protect the anaesthetic hands from injury. Systemic infection is treated by chemotherapy. Reconstructive surgery using tendon transfers may have a place even in the hand with sensory impairment.

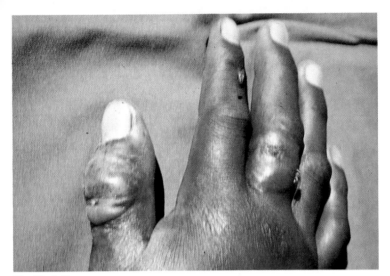

Fig. 89 Anthrax.

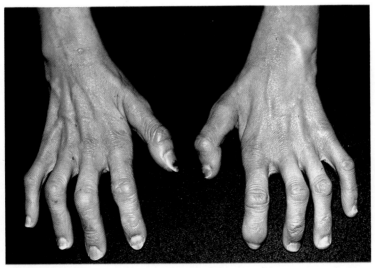

Fig. 90 Leprosy.

| # Benign Tumours (1)

Included under this heading are some lesions that are not true neoplasms but which present as swellings in the hand.

Ganglion

Incidence

Most common hand tumour.

Pathology

A cystic lesion with a fibrous capsule. It contains viscous material similar to synovial fluid.

Aetiology

May be caused by herniation of synovial tissue from a joint or be a form of mucoid degeneration of fibrous tissue.

Clinical features

Peak incidence in young adults. The most common site is the dorsal aspect of the wrist (Fig. 91) but they also occur on the volar aspect of the wrist, in association with the fibrous flexor sheaths, or as cysts within carpal bones.

Treatment

Fifty per cent disappear spontaneously. Treatment is indicated if the lesion increases in size or causes discomfort or pressure on a peripheral nerve. Rupture of the ganglion by pressure on injection is often followed by recurrence. Surgical excision, which should be carried out under tourniquet control with adequate anaesthesia, is more successful.

Inclusion dermoid

Incidence

Common.

Pathology

The subcutaneous implantation of a piece of skin results in a cyst lined with squamous epithelium and filled with keratin and sometimes cholesterol-rich fluid.

Aetiology

Trivial puncture wounds. Common in wire workers.

Clinical features

Firm swelling on volar aspect of hand (Fig. 92). Painless.

Treatment

Excision.

HAND CONDITIONS

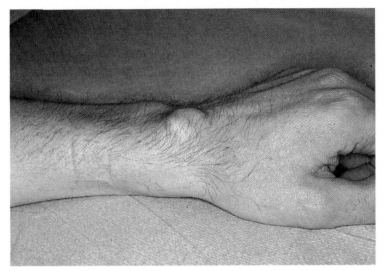

Fig. 91 Ganglion.

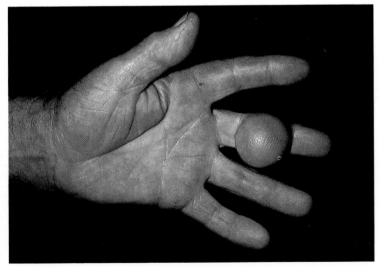

Fig. 92 Inclusion dermoid. This lesion is unusually large.

Benign Tumours (2)

Lipoma

Incidence Uncommon (about 5% of all hand tumours).

Pathology Proliferation of fat cells.

Clinical features A painless, smooth, soft swelling, usually in the palm of the hand (Fig. 93). More common in middle age. In some cases the lesion may be intraneural, the median nerve being a well-recognised site.

Treatment By surgical removal. Subcutaneous lesions can be shelled out by blunt dissection; intraneural·lesions can usually be dissected out under magnification.

Pigmented nodular synovitis

Also known as giant cell tumour of tendon sheath, fibrous xanthoma of synovium and pigmented nodular tenosynovitis.

Incidence Fairly common.

Pathology May be a true tumour or a reaction to injury or infection. The tumour is greyish and often contains yellow areas due to lipid and haemosiderin deposition. Histologically the lesion contains histiocytes and giant cells.

Clinical features More common in middle age. A painless, soft swelling on the flexor aspect of the fingers. Quite often the terminal interphalangeal joint is involved and the lesion may then be in a dorsal position (Fig. 94).

Treatment Excision. Recurrence may follow incomplete excision.

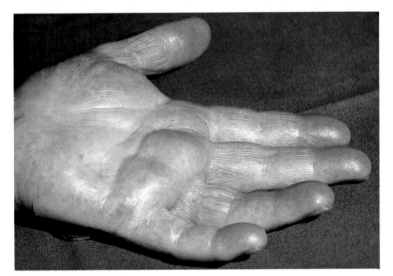

Fig. 93 Lipoma of palm.

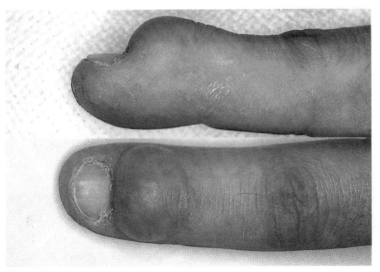

Fig. 94 Pigmented nodular synovitis.

Glomus tumour

Incidence

Uncommon.

Pathology

A well-defined, encapsulated lesion. It is derived from a glomus body, a collection of anastomosing blood vessels surrounded by nerves and epitheloid cells. Histologically the tumour is highly vascular and contains many nerve endings.

Clinical features

The patient complains of an exquisitely tender area at the tip of a finger which is extremely sensitive to heat and cold. Fifty per cent of glomus tumours are subungual. There is often no visible abnormality on clinical examination but a purplish lesion may be visible under the nail (Fig. 95). Delayed diagnosis is common. Radiographs sometimes show scalloping of the terminal phalanx (Fig. 96) — a common appearance when there is any tumour at the tip of the finger.

Treatment

Excision. Recurrence will take place if the tumour is not wholly removed.

Aneurysm

Incidence

Uncommon.

Pathology

Usually a false aneurysm or 'pulsating haematoma'. The ulnar artery or one of its branches is most often affected (Fig. 97). Usually there is a history of injury, such as repeatedly striking objects with the palm of the hand.

Clinical features

An ill-defined swelling in the hypothenar region, often pain-free and seldom pulsatile. The overlying skin may be red or bruised.

Treatment

Excision, after ensuring that the radial artery is providing an adequate blood supply.

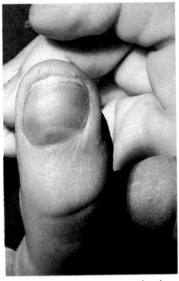

Fig. 95 A glomus tumour under the thumb nail.

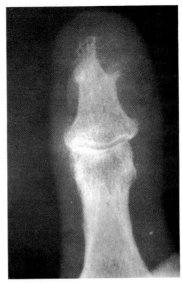

Fig. 96 Scalloping of the terminal phalanx.

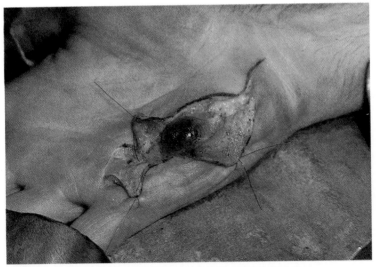

Fig. 97 A false aneurysm of the ulnar artery exposed at operation.

Enchondroma

Most common bone tumour in the hand. Half of all enchondromata are found in the hand.

Pathology

Usually solitary but are multiple in Ollier's disease (p. 49). The phalanges and the metacarpal bones are the most common sites. They are thought to arise from cartilage cells left behind during growth. They are usually centrally placed in the bone, but may be eccentrically placed (an ecchondroma). They do not increase in size when skeletal growth has ended and malignant change is very rare in single enchondromata.

Clinical features

May present as a hard, painless swelling (Fig. 98) or as a pathological fracture (Fig. 99), usually in adolescence. Radiographs show a circumscribed lytic lesion expanding the bone and containing irregular flecks of calcification.

Treatment

No treatment needed for asymptomatic lesions but they should be kept under radiographic review. If the lesion is large and unsightly or the diagnosis is in doubt curettage or excision should be performed, with bone grafting as necessary. Fractures through enchondromata heal well and definitive treatment of the tumour should await healing.

Exostosis

Pathology

Uncommon in hand and usually represents an osteochondroma.

Clinical features

A hard, painless, bony lump, usually fairly small (Fig. 100). Radiographs show a bony outgrowth.

Treatment

Excise if unsightly.

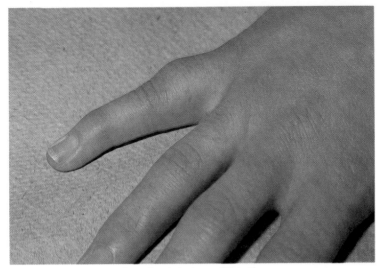

Fig. 98 Enchondroma of proximal phalanx of little finger.

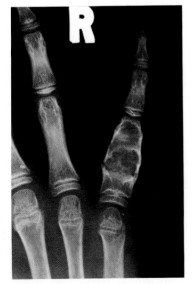

Fig. 99 A fracture through an enchondroma.

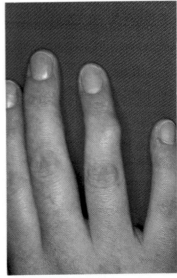

Fig. 100 Small exostosis on the intermediate phalanx.

16 | Malignant Tumours

Squamous carcinoma

Most common malignant tumour in the hand. Aetiological factors include excessive exposure to sunlight, X-rays and agents such as coal tar and oils.

Clinical features

Most common the back of the hand (Fig. 101). The tumour is an ulcerative or cauliflower-like lesion that may arise in an area of hyperkeratosis. Spread to regional nodes occurs in about 15%.

Treatment

Wide excision and skin grafting, or radiotherapy.

Malignant melanoma

This tumour of melanocytes is relatively uncommon.

Clinical features

Commoner in middle age. The lesion may be pigmented or amelanotic. The thumb is the most common site in the hand and tumour may be subungual or in the nail fold (Fig. 102). It may present as a chronic infected lesion, resistant to antibiotic treatment. Local and distant spread is common and occurs early.

Treatment

Excision biopsy followed by amputation of the affected digit. Immuno-, radio- and chemotherapy may be used in conjunction.

Chondrosarcoma

Fairly rare, but the most common malignant bone tumour in the hand.

Clinical features

About half arise in pre-existing cartilaginous tumours such as enchondromata (p. 71) or Ollier's disease (p. 49). They present as an expanding mass in the hand (Fig. 103). Metastases occur late.

Treatment

Total excision has a high cure rate.

HAND CONDITIONS

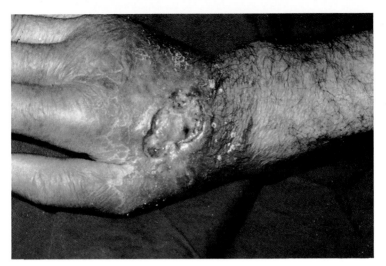

Fig. 101 Squamous carcinoma.

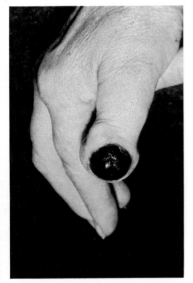

Fig. 102 Malignant melanoma.

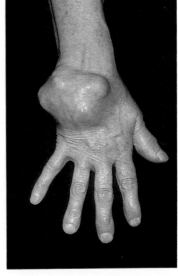

Fig. 103 Chondrosarcoma.

A common disorder in which the palmar and digital fascia becomes thickened and sometimes contracted.

Aetiological factors

Common in people of European descent but exceptionally rare in other races. There is a strong hereditary element and a predisposition to the disorder is transmitted as an autosomal dominant with variable penetrance. The condition is associated with other diseases such as epilepsy, cirrhosis of the liver and alcoholism, but such associations may not be of great significance as Dupuytren's disease is so common, occurring in 25% of men over the age of 65. It is not caused by injury, but injury may accelerate the onset of disease in those predisposed to it.

Pathology

Aggregates of contractile fibroblasts form in the palmar fascia and fascial planes of the fingers. Increased mitosis is present in the active phase.

Clinical features

It is a disease of middle and old age, but may occasionally affect young people. The common early presentation is with thickening or nodules in the palmar fascia (Fig. 104) without contracture. If the disease progresses to contracture the patient complains of inability to extend the finger. The palmar fascia on the ulnar side of the hand is most often affected and the ring finger and little fingers are most often involved (Fig. 105).

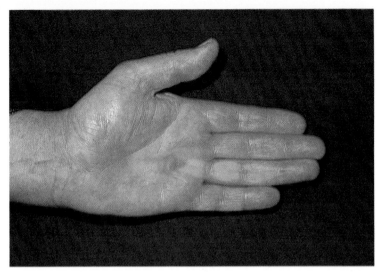

Fig. 104 Dupuytren's disease. There is a palmar nodule but no contracture.

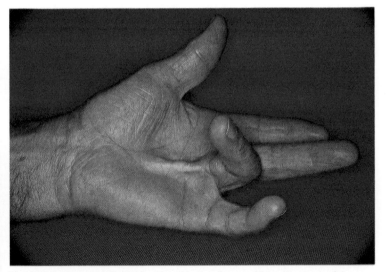

Fig. 105 Palmar and digital band to the ring finger with contracture of the metacarpophalangeal joint.

Knuckle pads, often tender, may be found on the dorsum of the proximal interphalangeal joints (Fig. 106) without evidence of Dupuytren's disease elsewhere; in those with a strong predisposition to the disease they may occur in young adult life.

Treatment

Treatment depends on the severity and progress of the disease. Knuckle pads and palmar thickening without contracture do not need treatment. Contractures may be static or increasing and their progress is frequently unpredictable. If there is a significant contracture or a small but increasing contracture, then treatment is indicated. Exercise and massage have no effect on the rate of increase in contracture. Fasciectomy (excision of the involved fascia) is the treatment of choice; fasciotomy (simple division of the band) or injections into the band give unsatisfactory results.

It is almost always possible to correct completely a contracture at the metacarpo-phalangeal joint by surgery. However, if the interphalangeal joints are affected (Fig. 107), secondary contractures in the ligaments of the joint (p. 3) usually prevent full correction of the deformity, even when all the affected fascia has been removed.

When there is very severe involvement or recurrence (Fig. 108) amputation of markedly contracted fingers may be warranted.

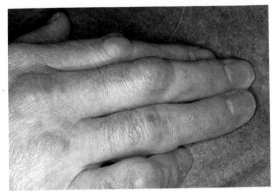

Fig. 106 Knuckle pads.

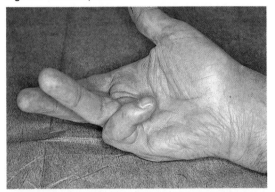

Fig. 107 Contractures at metacarpophalangeal and interphalangeal joints.

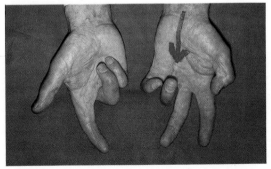

Fig. 108 Severe bilateral involvement. This patient had had several surgical procedures over many years for recurrent disease.

18 | Rheumatoid Arthritis (1)

An inflammatory arthropathy of unknown aetiology. It typically affects small joints in a symmetrical fashion at first, but larger joints may be affected in chronic sufferers.

Incidence

Common. More frequent in young and middle-aged women.

Pathology

The synovium is proliferative, producing swelling of joints, stretching of ligaments and damage to tendons. Articular cartilage is covered with a pannus that destroys the joint surface.

Clinical features

The small joints of the hand are often affected initially. The typical features are pain, swelling and stiffness. Thickened synovium may be palpated in the flexor compartment of the finger by the 'pinch test' (Fig. 109). Systemic symptoms such as malaise, weakness and loss of weight are often present.

Progression of the disease can lead to gross damage to the joints and soft tissues of the hand leaving a deformed hand with poor function (Fig. 110).

Treatment

Initially by anti-inflammatory and analgesic drugs, rest and splintage.

Surgical treatment aims to restore function rather than improve the appearance of the hand. Very careful assessment of the patient as a whole is needed before embarking on surgical treatment.

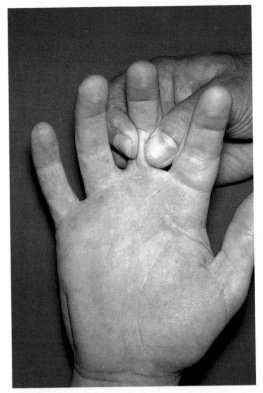

Fig. 109 The pinch test: in the normal subject (shown here) a fold of skin can easily be rolled between the examiner's fingers. When the test is positive a boggy swelling is felt.

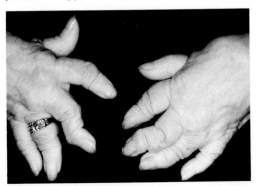

Fig. 110 Grossly deformed hands in late progressive rheumatoid arthritis.

Ulnar drift

Ulnar deviation of the fingers is one of the classical deformities in the rheumatoid hand (Fig. 111). Its pathogenesis is complex but it is partly attributable to synovitis in the metacarpophalangeal joints which stretches the collateral ligaments and causes displacement of the extensor tendons to the ulnar side of the metacarpal heads; contracture of the intrinsic muscles, common in rheumatoid arthritis, may also play a role.

Corrective surgery is directed towards obtaining stability at the metacarpophalangeal joints (which may require the use of artifical joints if there has been much destruction) and bringing the tendons back into their correct line of pull.

Z-deformity of thumb

The thumb is held flexed at the metacarpophalangeal joint and extended at the interphalangeal joint (Fig. 112). An adduction contracture of the first web space may also be present. The deformity is the result of arthritic changes in the metacarpophalangeal joint affecting the action of the extensor tendons and intrinsic muscles acting on the thumb. Stabilisation of the metacarpophalangeal joint will often improve the function of the thumb.

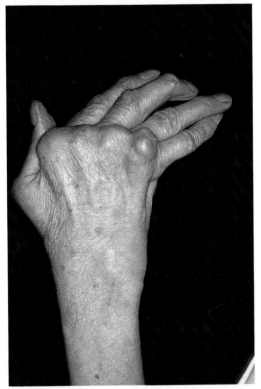

Fig. 111 Ulnar deviation of fingers.

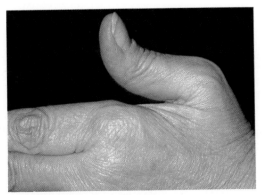

Fig. 112 Z-deformity of thumb.

18 | Rheumatoid Arthritis (3)

Swan neck deformity

The finger is held in hyperextension at the proximal interphalangeal joint and flexion at the distal interphalangeal joint (Fig. 113). Like most rheumatoid deformities it is the result of imbalance in the actions of muscles which follows the destruction of joints and stretching of ligaments and tendons by proliferative synovium. A swan neck deformity may follow rupture or stretching of the extensor tendon on the dorsum of the distal interphalangeal joint, initially producing a mallet finger deformity (p. 21). It may also be secondary to stretching of the volar plate of the proximal interphalangeal joint. It is a fairly constant 'rule' that in rheumatoid arthritis the joints adjacent to a deformed joint tend to develop the opposite deformity.

Boutonnière deformity

The finger is held in flexion at the proximal interphalangeal joint and hyperextension at the distal interphalangeal joint (Fig. 114). The pathogenesis of this deformity is described on page 21. In rheumatoid arthritis the central slip of the extensor tendon is damaged on the dorsum of the proximal interphalangeal joint by proliferative synovium arising from the joint.

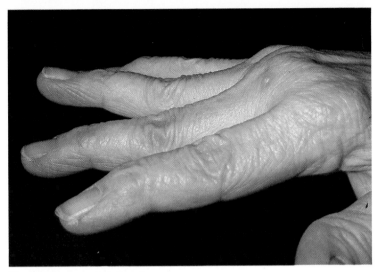

Fig. 113 Swan neck deformity.

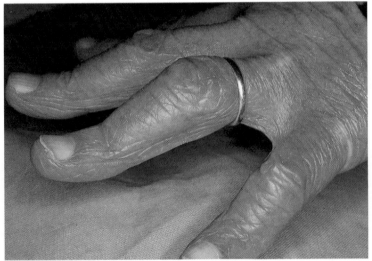

Fig. 114 Boutonnière deformity.

Dorsal synovitis

The wrist is frequently affected by the inflammatory processes of rheumatoid arthritis. Proliferative synovium arises from the synovial sheaths around tendons and the wrist joint itself. The abnormal synovium on the dorsum of the wrist is usually visible and palpable. A constriction in the middle of the swelling caused by the extensor retinaculum results in an 'hourglass' appearance (Fig. 115).

Pain on extending the fingers and thumb in the presence of dorsal synovitis is an indication that rupture of the extensor tendons is impending; surgical decompression or removal of the synovium may be necessary to prevent this.

Rupture of extensor tendons

Rupture of the extensor tendons more often occurs in those running across the ulnar part of the wrist (Fig. 116). The tendons may be damaged by synovial proliferation or by attrition on the head of the ulna which is commonly subluxated dorsally. Excision of the head of the ulna and reconstruction of the tendons may be necessary to relieve pain and restore function.

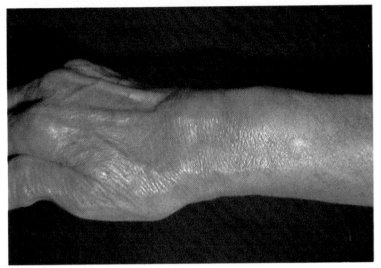

Fig. 115 Proliferative synovium under the extensor retinaculum.

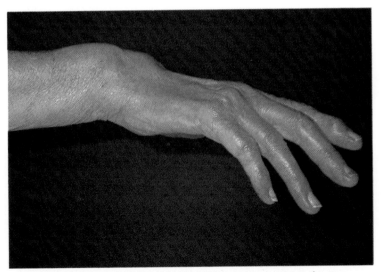

Fig. 116 Rupture of the extensor tendons. The patient is attempting to straighten her fingers.

Osteoarthritis (1)

Although primary osteoarthritis usually affects large weight-bearing joints such as the hip it is not uncommon in the hand although the symptoms and disability may be slight.

Heberden's nodes

Clinical features

Small bony lumps at the terminal interphalangeal joints of the fingers (Fig. 117). They are related to the formation of osteophytes and may commence with redness and pain around the joint which settles after a few months.

Treatment

Pain and stiffness usually respond to analgesics; if pain is severe surgical fusion of the joint may be necessary.

Mucous cyst

Clinical features

A cystic swelling arising from the dorsum of an osteoarthritic terminal interphalangeal joint (Fig. 118). It may arise from either side of the extensor tendon and typically lies between the joint line and the nail fold. Mucous cysts are prone to become infected and may drain synovial fluid.

Treatment

Excise only if large and unsightly; recurrence and/or discharging sinus are frequent after operation. Local rotational skin flaps may be necessary to close a defect over the joint.

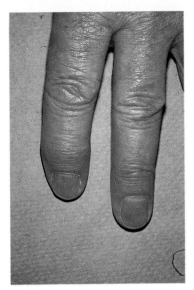

Fig. 117 Heberden's nodes.

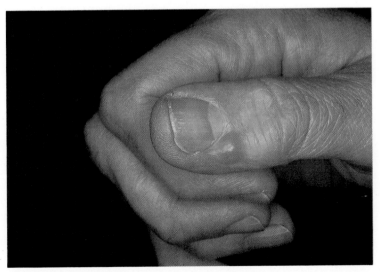

Fig. 118 Mucous cyst of interphalangeal joint of thumb.

19 | Osteoarthritis (2)

Carpometacarpal joint of thumb

This is a common site for primary osteoarthritis.

Clinical features

Not always symptomatic. However, there may be local pain, especially on gripping, and an adduction contracture of the thumb may develop.

Radiological features

Loss of articular cartilage, sclerosis of bones adjacent to the joint and the formation of osteophytes (Fig. 119).

Treatment

Surgery is reserved for those who have not responded to conservative treatment. Various operations are in use, including excision of the trapezium, with or without prosthetic replacement and fusion of the joint.

20 | Gout

A metabolic disorder in which there is deposition of monosodium urate in the tissues.

Clinical features

Sudden onset of pain, swelling and redness, usually affecting joints in the foot or the knee, but the hand is not infrequently affected (Fig. 120). Gout affecting the fingers is often misdiagnosed as an infection such as paronychia; the diagnosis of gout is supported by a raised level of serum urate.

Treatment

Acute symptoms controlled by an anti-inflammatory drug such as phenylbutazone; long term treatment with a uricosuric agent is necessary.

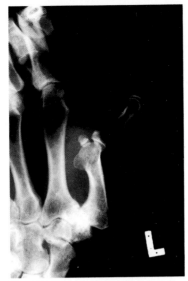

Fig. 119 Osteoarthritis affecting the trapeziometacarpal joint of the thumb.

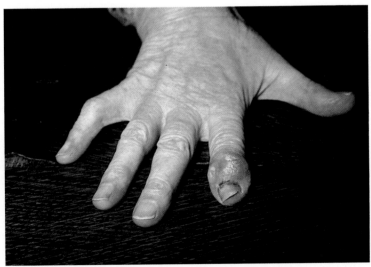

Fig. 120 Acute gout affecting the terminal interphalangeal joint.

Skin Diseases (1)

Psoriasis

A common, chronic skin disorder of unknown aetiology, characterised by raised, red, scaly patches of varying size; it may be associated with nail changes and damage to the joints in the hand.

Clinical features

The typical feature in the hand is pitting of the nail, which may or may not be found in association with the skin changes of psoriasis (Fig. 121).

Psoriatic arthropathy affects the small joints of the hand. There is often marked destruction and severe deformity that may be sudden in onset and rapid in progression (Fig. 122). Arthropathy occurs in about 10% of those affected by psoriasis; the skin changes may be unimpressive even when the arthopathy is severe, but it is rare for joint changes to precede skin manifestations.

Treatment

Nail pitting may improve if the skin responds to treatment with dermatological preparation, but the arthropathy is unaffected. Joint disease is treated with anti-inflammatory drugs; surgical fusion of unstable joints may be necessary if destruction is severe.

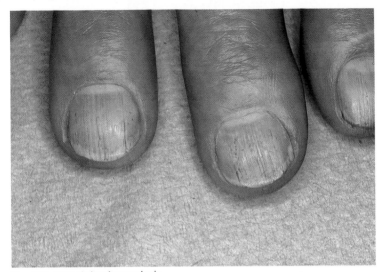

Fig. 121 Nail pitting in psoriasis.

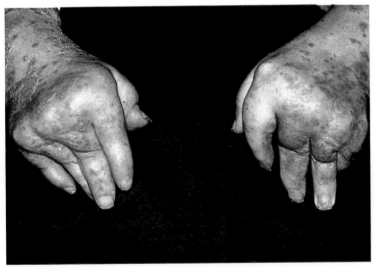

Fig. 122 Psoriatic arthropathy. This patient has florid skin changes of psoriasis.

Eczema

A non-infective inflammatory disorder of the skin. It may be due to external irritants (contact dermatitis) but is frequently a reaction pattern to unknown stimuli (endogenous dermatitis). The hand is a common site for either main group.

Aetiology

Contact dermatitis: usually a history of exposure to some irritant but careful detective work may be necessary to identify it. Endogenous type: unknown, but hereditary, immunological, emotion, infective and vasomotor factors may all play a part.

Clinical features

Extremely variable. In contact dermatitis itching, redness and blistering occur (Fig. 123). Endogenous eczema may commence in a similar way with an itchy vesicular rash, but in the chronic phase the epidermis is thickened and oedematous with prominent skin lines. Secondary skin infection can occur in both types.

Treatment

Protection from the irritant substance(s) will prevent recurrence of contact dermatitis. In more chronic forms zinc and salicylate paste and steroid lotions are the mainstays of treatment.

Vitiligo

Absence of skin pigmentation.

Aetiology

Unknown. An autoimmune response may be involved.

Clinical features

Appears in patches on face, backs of hands (Fig. 124), axillae and perineum in childhood or later life.

Treatment

Unsatisfactory. Locally injected steroids may have some effect. Cosmetic camouflage cream is useful.

HAND CONDITIONS

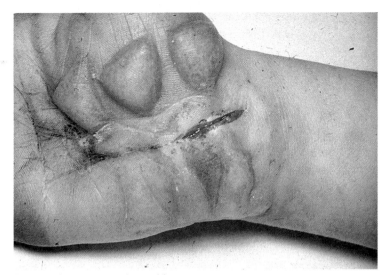

Fig. 123 Acute contact dermatitis.

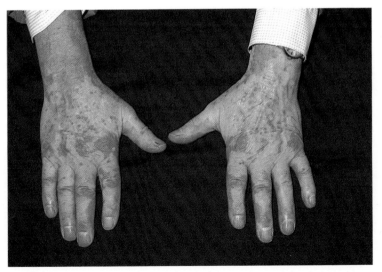

Fig. 124 Vitiligo.

Scleroderma

A collagen disorder characterised by sclerosis of the skin and alimentary tract, heart and lungs.

Aetiology
Unknown.

Pathology
Fibrosis of affected structures associated with obliterative vascular changes.

Clinical features
Women are affected much more commonly than men. Frank scleroderma may be preceded by Raynaud's disease, a painful condition affecting young women in which the fingers show abnormal vasoconstriction in response to cold. Scleroderma affecting the hands (sclerodactyly) results in vasomotor disturbances, thickening and hardening of the skin, trophic changes (Fig. 125) and nodules of subcutaneous calcification (Fig. 126). Visceral sclerosis tends to be delayed in this type of scleroderma.

Treatment
Symptomatic. Surgical removal of the calcified nodules is sometimes necessary.

Acrocyanosis

Persistent cyanosis in the hands of young women without evidence of organic vascular disease (Fig. 127).

Aetiology
Unknown. Sometimes familial.

Clinical features
The cyanosis is worse in cold weather but it is painless and not associated with trophic changes.

Treatment
Reassurance. Keep hands warm.

HAND CONDITIONS

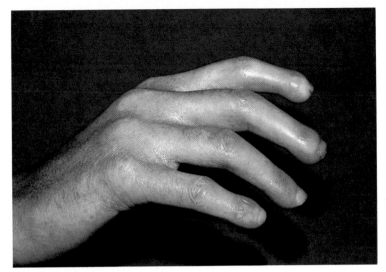

Fig. 125 Scleroderma.

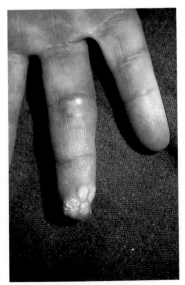

Fig. 126 Calcified nodules in scleroderma.

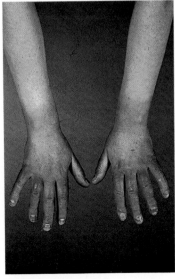

Fig. 127 Acrocyanosis.

23 | Carpal Tunnel Syndrome

A disorder caused by compression of the median nerve in the carpal tunnel beneath the flexor retinaculum at the wrist.

Incidence

Common, especially in middle-aged women.

Aetiology

Frequently idiopathic, but may be associated with rheumatoid arthritis, fluid retention during pregnancy or any anatomical abnormality or tumour occupying space in the carpal tunnel.

Clinical features

Typically the patient is woken during the night by a pain described as 'burning' or 'bursting'. The pain may not be confined to the median nerve distribution; often the whole hand and forearm are affected. The discomfort is relieved by some activity such as shaking the hand, running cold water over it, or getting up and making tea. The hand may feel heavy and numb in the mornings.

On examination there is often no abnormality and only in advanced cases is median nerve paresis detectable clinically. Unforced flexion of the wrist for about a minute reproduces the symptoms in about 75% of patients (Phalen's test — Fig. 128).

Treatment

Conservative: by splinting the wrist, diuretic drugs or injection of hydrocortisone into the carpal tunnel.
Surgical: decompression of the carpal tunnel (Fig. 129) is very successful.

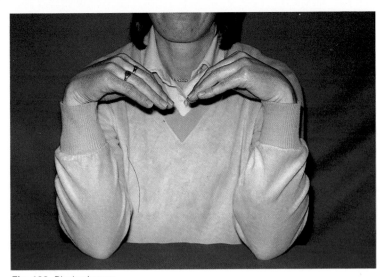

Fig. 128 Phalen's test.

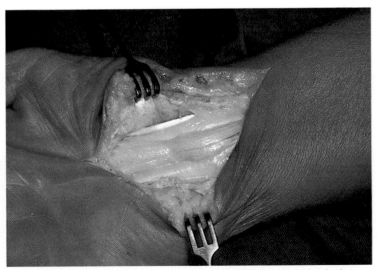

Fig. 129 Decompression of the carpal tunnel. Note the constriction in the median nerve.

| # Stenosing Tenosynovitis

De Quervain's tenosynovitis

An inflammatory, constricting synovitis of the first dorsal compartment of the wrist through which run the tendons of extensor pollicis brevis and abductor pollicis longus.

Aetiology

Uncertain, but may be related to repetitious movements.

Clinical features

Commonly affects middle-aged women. There is pain at the radial styloid process, aggravated by gripping when the wrist is ulnar deviated; this may cause heavy objects such as teapots to be dropped.

The thickened fibrous sheath may be palpable. Passive ulnar deviation of the wrist with the thumb gripped in the palm often reproduces the pain (Finkelstein's test — Fig. 130).

Treatment

Conservative: splintage or injection of hydrocortisone into the affected compartment. *Surgical:* decompression of the compartment. It is important to avoid injury to terminal branches of the radial nerve.

Trigger finger

A common condition in which a finger or thumb sticks in the flexed position (Fig. 131). The fibrous flexor sheath may be narrowed or the tendon enlarged, for example by a rheumatoid nodule.

Clinical features

The digit must be straightened passively by the patient and this is associated with some discomfort.

Treatment

Surgical decompression of the mouth of the flexor tendon sheath, or local injection of hydrocortisone. Injection should be avoided if the tendon is thought to be abnormal as it may precipitate rupture.

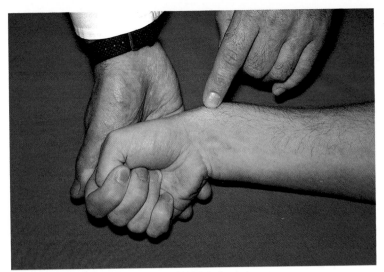

Fig. 130 De Quervain's tenosynovitis. Finkelstein's test.

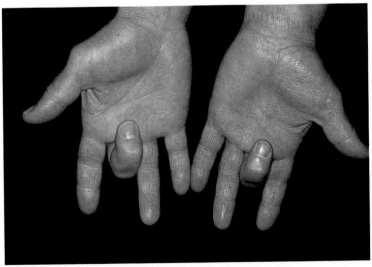

Fig. 131 Trigger finger. The typical position of flexion.

25 | Volkmann's Contracture

Ischaemic fibrosis of the forearm muscles, most commonly after a supracondylar fracture of the humerus in children.

Pathology

Interruption of the arterial supply or venous drainage causes ischaemic swelling of the muscles in their fascial compartments and further obstruction to the microcirculation.

Clinical features

The flexor compartment is usually affected. Following reduction of the fracture there is severe and increasing pain, aggravated by passive extension of the fingers. In the late untreated case fibrosis of muscles and ischaemic nerve damage produces a claw hand and flexion of the wrist (Fig. 132).

Treatment

Early: release tight bandages and gently extend the elbow; if no response the deep fascia should be released without delay. *Late:* splintage and reconstructive surgery may improve function.

26 | Cerebral Palsy

A group of chronic non-progressive brain disorders which cause impaired motor function.

Clinical features

Muscle tone, power and co-ordination are affected to a variable degree. If the hand is affected it may be held in an abnormal posture (Fig. 133).

Treatment

In some patients hand function can be improved by splintage, stabilisation procedures and tendon transfers.

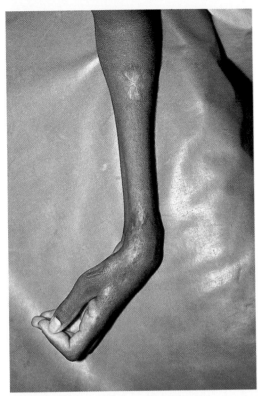

Fig. 132 Volkmann's ischaemic contracture.

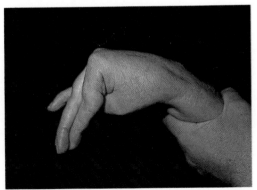

Fig. 133 Abnormal posture of the hand in cerebral palsy. Note the 'thumb in palm' deformity.

See also glomus tumour (p. 69), melanoma (p. 73) and psoriasis (p. 91).

Splinter haemorrhages

A common lesion.

Clinical appearance

They are seen as small red streaks lying beneath the nail with their long axes parallel to that of the nail (Fig. 134).

Causes

Classically they are associated with subacute bacterial endocarditis, but they may also be seen in minor trauma, rheumatoid arthritis, psoriasis, dermatitis, fungal infections and in the presence of mitral stenosis. Since they are found in so many different conditions they are not of great diagnostic value.

Fungal infections

Common. *Trichophyton rubrum* is the fungus most often isolated.

Clinical features

Affected nails become thickened, cracked and discoloured (Fig. 135). Part of the nail may break away. Fungi can be identified on specially prepared nail clippings.

Treatment

Local treatments do not influence the infection because it is deep in the nail and its bed. Systemic griseofulvin is highly effective.

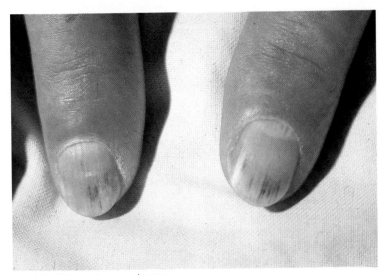

Fig. 134 Splinter haemorrhages.

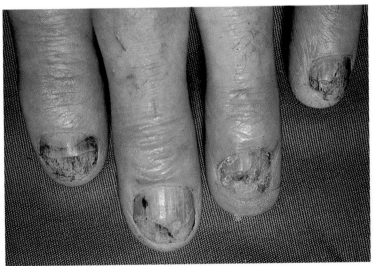

Fig. 135 Fungal infection of nails.

Nail Disorders (2)

Beau's lines

Clinical appearance

Seen as a depression across the surface of all nails. In severe cases the nails may be shed (Fig. 136).

Causes

The lines are caused by severe illnesses in which nail growth ceases. The nail changes are seen some weeks later when nail growth has recommenced.

Beau's lines are typically seen after coronary thrombosis, severe chest infection and, in children, measles.

Clubbing

Clinical appearance

Loss of the normal angle between the nail and the nail fold (Fig. 137). All nails are affected.

Causes

The mechanism of production is uncertain, but it is possibly related to increased blood flow and soft tissue proliferation in the terminal phalanges.

Clubbing typically occurs in lung or heart diseases associated with cyanosis. It may also be seen in thyroid disease, biliary cirrhosis and bowel disorders such as sprue and ulcerative colitis; occasionally it is idiopathic.

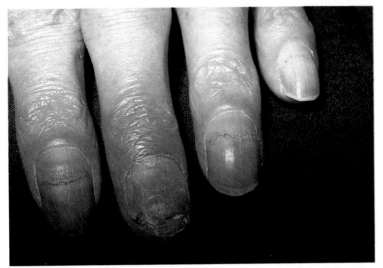

Fig. 136 Beau's lines in a patient who had had a severe chest infection some weeks before.

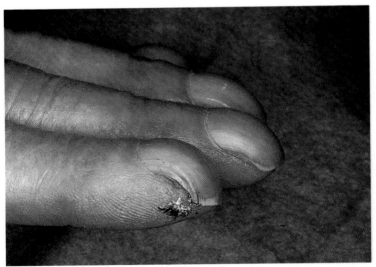

Fig. 137 Clubbing.